THE CAREGIVER'S
GUIDE TO
WOUND CARE

THE CAREGIVER'S
GUIDE TO
WOUND CARE

Jennifer J. Taylor, MD

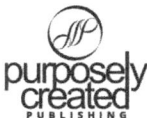

purposely
created
PUBLISHING

A CAREGIVER'S GUIDE TO WOUND CARE
Published by Purposely Created Publishing Group™
Copyright © 2018 Jennifer Taylor

All rights reserved.

Printed in the United States of America

ISBN: 978-1-948400-59-6

Special discounts are available on bulk quantity purchases by book clubs, associations and special interest groups. For details email: sales@publishyourgift.com or call (888) 949-6228.

For information logon to: www.PublishYourGift.com

Dedication

This book is dedicated to my patients, the ones who trusted me with their limbs and lives. It is also dedicated to every caregiver out there, silently struggling to handle the overwhelming needs of loved ones who are no longer able to care for themselves. Walking this path is both difficult and demanding, and I salute you for your sacrifice.

A special thanks to every wound care nurse I've ever worked with. You guys are absolutely awesome! I am forever grateful for all that you've taught me.

Sharon, Sue, Kathy, and Nina and the entire Vista crew: thanks for your patience and for the laughs. I really miss you guys!

I've also had the pleasure of working with some stellar podiatrists, vascular surgeons, and wound-care physicians as well. Let's continue healing the world, one wound at a time.

Finally, a huge thank you to my family because, without you, I literally would not be who I am. Thank you for believing in me. Taryn and Cameron, you are the greatest loves of my life. Thank you for keeping a smile on my face with your humor and playfulness.

Table of Contents

Introduction

I have a passion for wound care. I thrive on taking a patient from being wounded to healed through my actions, decisions, teaching, and care. I absolutely love draining pus collections, cutting away dead tissue, and stitching up injuries. I get excited about clean, healthy tissue in a wound bed. Even after many years of training and practice, I'm still fascinated by the human body. Nothing excites or challenges me more than figuring out why a wound won't heal and thinking of new approaches to get it to close. Odd as it may be, treating wounds is my calling.

It grieves me when I find people who have suffered from unhealed wounds for years and have given up any hope for healing. Tragically, literally millions of people in the U.S. undergo limb amputations that might've been prevented if only they had received the proper wound care.

I was first introduced to wound care while I was working as a hospice physician in Central Illinois. I found myself at a loss when trying to come up with solutions to help my patients and their caregivers treat their wounds, because I had received very little training in wound care during my family medicine residency. The only thing that I knew to do was to cover wet wounds with a dry dressing and to change that dressing two to three times daily. Later on in my career, I learned how that basic treatment regimen was grossly inefficient and, in some cases, even harmful. From there, I underwent dedicated training in wound care and discovered one of the most essential elements in wound healing: proper moisture balance.

During this time, I noticed that my eczema was getting worse and that my hands were constantly dry, itchy, and irritated. My "go to" emollient-based lotion was no longer working, its formula no match for the harsh medical-grade soaps that I used throughout the day while caring for patients. I researched solutions online and discovered a few recipes for homemade moisturizers that contained only natural ingredients. I began experimenting with different combinations of butters such as shea, mango, and cocoa. I had learned through caring for all sorts of skin wounds that both too much and too little moisture injured the skin, and dyes and strong perfumes irritated it further. In fact, nursing home patients whose skin was moisturized and soft didn't have as many skin tears and injuries as patients whose skin remained dry.

Through trial and error, I found a combination of ingredients that worked well for my hands and for my then two-year-old grandson who was also suffering from widespread eczema. This hobby turned into a passion, and I ended up starting my own line of moisturizing skin products. I continue to coach caregivers on the basics of wound care in order to keep their loved ones' skin intact and injury free.

Speaking of caring for loved ones: let's face it, caregiving is hard. The hours are long, and the work is gritty. Your family member has twenty-four-hour needs that don't stop. Feeding, bathing, grooming, toileting, attending doctor appointments, managing medications, filling prescriptions—the list of things to do can seem endless. You take care of everyone else and, by the end of the day, you have very little time and energy left to tend to your own needs.

When your loved one has a skin wound, the situation can be even more challenging. The wound requires dressing changes, sometimes multiple times daily. Wounds are often quite painful too, especially if they get infected, and even the smallest ones can take months to resolve. The cost of supplies can also be a huge burden and barrier to healing. Perhaps your loved one's primary doctor never gave you affordable or satisfying treatment options to help with healing.

I'll let you in on a secret: most primary care physicians do not know how to take care of wounds or know that the field of wound care even exists. Wound care is not part of our training in medical school or residency, even though there have been many new, highly specialized developments in wound care and its treatment strategies. With everything that doctors have to learn about the human body and the thousands of diseases that we will encounter within a relatively short amount of time, wound care has yet to make its way up the list of medical education priorities. In my residency training, I was fortunate to have a few opportunities to care for chronic wounds, but many important details were glazed over. For instance, there was no teaching on the difference between a healthy and unhealthy wound, and the importance of removing unhealthy tissue from the wound bed was not stressed. This lack of knowledge and physician training in wound care contributes to prolonged suffering and worse patient outcomes.

Given this, you cannot always rely on your primary physician to recognize when your loved one's wound has become problematic and requires specialized care. It's up to you to be the advocate for your family member.

In this book, we'll explore ways to prevent your loved one from getting skin wounds and learn practical tips on how to treat open wounds and get them to heal. This crash course will help you understand the basics of wound care so that caring for your loved one's skin will be less of a guessing game. It will also help you understand when you need to get a wound care specialist involved and how to ask the right questions when the time comes.

I will introduce some technical terms with clear, plain explanations, instead of the "Medicalese" that we physicians use all too often. This will allow you to articulate some of the language used in wound care and communicate better with your wound care team. Sometimes, using the technical terms can't be avoided, so I've also included a glossary at the end of the book. Don't be afraid to flip back to it and refresh your memory on what a particular term means if you're unsure or have simply forgotten.

I hope that this book will be a resource for you to refer back to when you get stuck in caring for your loved one!

1

What Is a Chronic Wound?

Before we can talk about what a chronic wound is and how it gets to that state, we need to spend a few moments discussing the normal healing process. I'll try to keep this short and sweet—or at least not too painful. Here we go!

Normally, it takes about twenty-one days for a skin injury to heal. A wound is considered chronic when it hasn't healed in about two to three months. During the typical three weeks to three months after an injury, there are a number of phases that the skin goes through on the path to restoration. The first thing that happens at the time of injury is hemostasis: blood vessels constrict (clamp down or narrow) to stop any bleeding. Platelets, a type of blood cell, arrive on the scene of injury and, along with a protein called fibrin, seal off the bleeding. This is similar to the way you'd patch a leaking water hose.

The second phase is inflammation. During this time, fluid leaks out from the cells of the injured tissue, healing cells come in, and damaged cells get removed. This phase is painful because some of the healing proteins that get released can cause pain. Swelling also occurs. Even so, inflammation is a natural response to injury; in fact, we need inflammation to protect us during the healing process.

The third phase of the normal healing process is proliferation. In this stage, new cells made of collagen and other proteins begin to grow, and new blood vessels develop in order to supply the tissue with oxygen and vital nutrients. The collagen, proteins, and new blood vessels form a substance called granulation tissue. We get excited about seeing granulation tissue in a wound because it is a sign that the skin is healing. The wound then contracts (gets smaller), the new epithelial (skin) cells grow in from the edges of the wound and on top of the granulation tissue, and the gap is filled.

The final phase is maturation. You can't see this phase happening, but during this time, the collagen finishes transforming, the body absorbs all the excess fluid it created, the swelling goes away, and the wound fully closes. This phase can take as long as a year to finish, even though with the naked eye, it looks as if it's already complete. Unfortunately, the skin is never as strong as it was before it was injured.

A wound becomes chronic when it gets stuck in any one of the four phases. The most common phase in which healing gets stuck is the inflammation stage. The problems start when this phase continues for too long or when the response is too powerful. Like calling the U. S. Army to come in and break up schoolyard fight between fourth graders, when your body calls in too

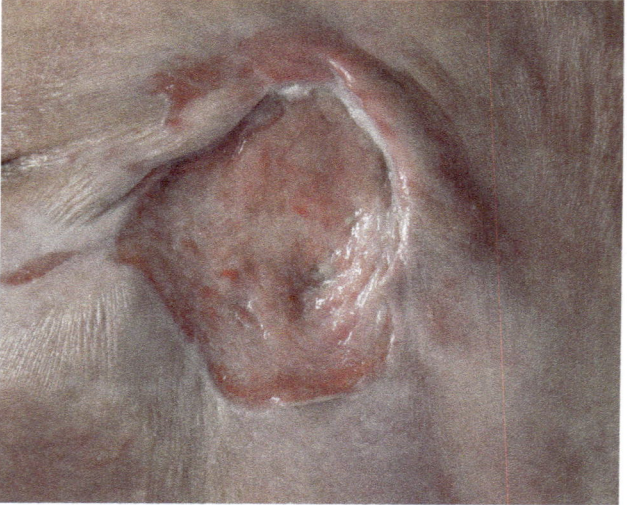

many inflammatory proteins for help, the response is way out of proportion to what is required, and the army of inflammatory proteins can end up causing more harm than good.

A wound becomes chronic when it gets stuck in any one of the four phases. The most common phase where healing gets stuck is the inflammation stage. But what makes a wound get stuck in the inflammatory phase? Often the cause is that the wound gets colonized with bacteria or infected, or that excess wound fluid that is released as a normal part of inflammation causes growth factors to get broken down. Without the growth factors, the wound cannot heal. When the inflammatory phase lasts too long, fibroblasts (another special type of proteins) that are necessary for healing get depleted so new tissue can't be made. Sometimes the very products we use on the skin in an attempt to cleanse or disinfect it turn out to stop the healing process because those products stop cell growth.

2

How Do Chronic Wounds Develop?

The skin can be injured in any number of ways. In terms of family members that are bedbound or have limited ability to move, the most common type of wound is a *pressure ulcer*, commonly known as a bed sore. A pressure ulcer is an injury to the skin caused by prolonged pressure against an external surface, including common household items such beds, wheelchairs, and pillows, and even our own bodies. Pressure ulcers happen on areas of skin that lie on top of bone, like the heels, spine, hips, ankles, knees, and shoulders.

Normally, when an area of your body has been in a position for too long, you start to feel uncomfortable, and this makes you move or shift your weight. If you are disabled, elderly, or otherwise weak and frail, you cannot shift your weight or change positions. The skin and tissue between your bone and the external surface get less blood and oxygen flow, so the tissue gets injured and begins to die. If the pressure is relieved in time, you may end up with a deep bruise; if not, the injury leads to an ulcer.

How can a pillow cause a pressure ulcer when pillows are soft? The answer is in your loved one's fragile skin, which is prone to injury. Long-term illness weakens the body's natural defenses and decreases its ability to withstand minor, everyday challenges. But because of conditions like poor circulation and diabetes, your loved one may not even notice the discomfort healthier people feel when they've been in one position for too long. They don't or can't change position, and the pressure gets prolonged. If prolonged, the pressure cuts off blood flow to the affected area, and the skin starts to die.

As mentioned earlier, pressure injuries range from getting a deep bruise to getting ulcers that travel through the layers of the skin, sometimes all the way into muscle. Those deep bruises are called deep tissue injury or DTI in the wound care world. You can tell a DTI apart from a superficial bruise because a DTI doesn't fade when you touch it; it stays discolored. When you touch your every-day bruise with your finger, the purple/blue/red color disappears and, when you remove your finger, it comes back. Also, an every-day bruise is gone within two to three days, while a DTI can take two to three weeks or longer to heal. And if pressure continues to be placed on a DTI, the injury will get deeper and more serious.

Another cause of skin wounds is *poor circulation*. There are two classes of wounds that fit under the category of poor circulation. First, when blood doesn't flow properly from the extremities and back toward the heart, the condition is called venous insufficiency. When you suffer this type of vein

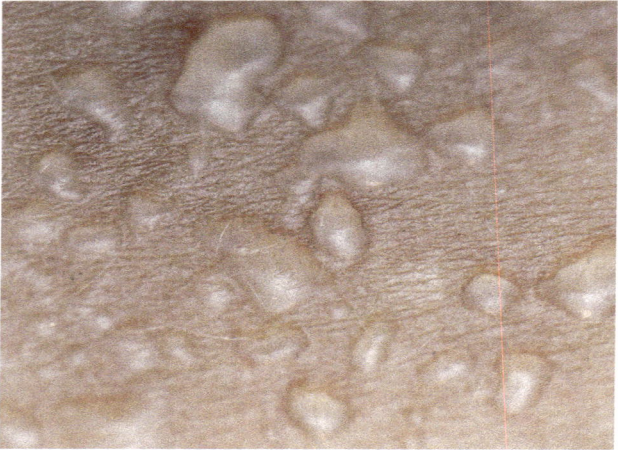

problem for a long time, wounds develop and, unfortunately, these are some of the hardest to treat. Basically, if fluid cannot get back to the heart, it pools in the legs, ankles, and feet, causing swelling (edema). When the legs get too swollen, the edema blocks blood flow to the skin and skin cells cannot renew themselves. Extra fluid then starts to leak out of the vessels and onto the skin's surface and the legs "weep." This fluid contains proteins that hurt the skin, weakening it and causing pain, discoloration, and heaviness in the legs. Because the skin is weakened, damaged, and not getting enough healthy blood flow, when minor injuries like bumping the leg or an incidental scratch occur, they cause a worse injury to the skin than they normally would and the injury is at a high risk of healing poorly or slowly.

The second class of wounds that stem from poor circulation is called arterial wounds, which occur when blood doesn't flow well from the heart to the extremities. Blood that comes from the heart is rich in oxygen and that oxygen is needed in every organ in the body including the skin, the body's largest organ. When our organs and tissues don't get enough oxygen, they begin to die. So, when diseases like high cholesterol and high blood pressure cause decreased blood flow in your body, the skin is also negatively affected. Wounds occur much more easily and then are slow to heal. Diseased arteries are the cause of many conditions like heart attacks, strokes, and gangrene, which leads to limb amputations.

Diabetes also causes skin wounds that are quite difficult to heal, especially when blood sugars are not controlled. Diabetic patients tend to have dry skin and, without the right amount of moisture, the skin's defenses are weakened. Diabetes can also damage collagen, which compromises the skin's structure and function.

Diabetes causes nerve damage called neuropathy, which is a condition where the nerves do not send and receive messages properly, thus the normal pain response to injury does not occur. Ordinary scratches and major insults like burns or punctures may go unnoticed by your diabetic family member, because they lose sensation over time and literally do not feel anything in their extremities. This is why it is important to check your loved one's feet for any thick callouses, scratches, or cracks in the skin that can provide an opening for germs to get in. In fact, calloused skin makes matter worse since it has less nerve endings on the surface, which means that feeling and reaction toward puncture is further decreased.

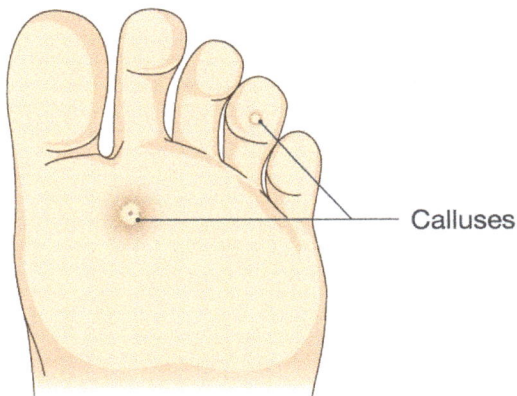

Calluses

Diabetic foot ulcers are one of the top causes of amputation in the U.S. They are often quite small and rather unimpressive in
how they look, but they have high potential to travel from the skin's surface into the
deeper tissues, including muscle and bone.
When deep wounds become infected, bone
infections can easily follow. Chronic osteomyelitis, a serious bone infection that does
not respond to antibiotics, is a frequent
precursor for amputation.

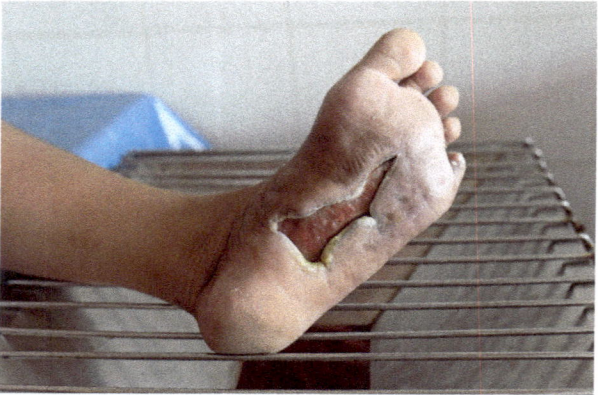

In order to avoid such serious situations, make sure your loved one wears non-skid socks or diabetic shoes whenever they are moving about, even if they are wheelchair bound. It is very common to injure toes, ankles, and heels even when one is moving about in a wheelchair.

Chapter

▼ 3

What Are Some Risk Factors for Chronic Wounds?

Let's go over some of the most common risks and lifestyle factors that may contribute to the development of chronic wounds. These are important to keep in mind considering that, as our skin weakens, trauma occurs more often and easily. If your loved one has serious risk factors, even surgical incisions are in danger of not healing properly.

Advanced Age

As we age, our skin ages too. So, what happens? We lose layers of fat and collagen that give our skin structure and protection. The rate of skin regeneration slows: instead of turning over new cells every twenty to twenty-five days, it takes closer to thirty to thirty-five days. The glands in our skin that make oil become less active, so, again, we lose that layer of protection. We also lose our ability to hold on to water, which is critical in maintaining healthy skin and growing new skin cells. Simply put, the skin becomes thinner, drier, and more fragile and can no longer protect us against injury the way it once did. Little bumps or scratches that you never used to pay much attention to can now cause tears or an open wound that take weeks or months to heal.

Poor Nutrition

Unfortunately, people with a lot of ongoing medical problems don't have strong appetites. As a result, they don't eat the right amount of vitamins, protein, healthy fats, and minerals, many of which are absolutely necessary for repairing skin damage. Examples include, but are not limited to, biotin, vitamin A, B, C, D, E, and K. Vitamin A and B5 increase the firmness of your skin and build moisture. Vitamins C and E act as antioxidants, which help to protect your skin and fight damage from the sun and other pollutants in the environment. Without these nutrients, the skin is easier to damage and slower to repair. You can help offset gaps in your loved one's diet by giving them vitamins and supplements. A word of caution though: too much vitamin A, D, E, and K can be deadly so just be careful not to buy supplements that have more than 100% of these particular vitamins. More is *not* always better.

Obesity

People who are severely overweight have an increased amount of skin injuries. When one area of skin remains in contact with another (such as the area underneath the breasts and underneath the belly), warmth and moisture increase. This is the perfect set-up for yeast infections because yeast thrives in a warm, moist environment. Infected skin is vulnerable skin.

Also, increased body surface area and depth of fat beneath the skin tax the body's demand for blood flow. There is simply more area to protect and the nutrient-and-oxygen-rich blood and healing cells that come from the heart must travel farther distances to get to their destination.

Uncontrolled Diabetes

This condition compromises your immune system and impairs your healing response. That's why bacterial skin infections like boils and folliculitis are more common in diabetics whose blood sugars are not controlled. Diabetes also causes damage to small and medium-sized blood vessels, which supply oxygen and nutrients to your skin. This results in a group of skin problems called dermopathy. Fungal infections of the nails, fingers, toes, and breasts are all much more common in diabetic patients.

Poor Blood Flow

Smoking, high blood pressure, and high

cholesterol all slow down your body's blood flow by constricting (narrowing) the blood vessels or by creating plaque on the inside the vessels. Think of it like a four-lane highway being reduced to a one-lane street lined with parked cars: the blood, which contains all the healing and repair proteins that your body needs to fix injuries, cannot readily get to the area where it's needed. This also means that oxygen cannot get delivered to your skin. Without it, your skin will die. No specialized dressing can change that. Nothing in our body can survive without oxygen—we've simply got to have it.

Compromised Immune System

Your immunes system can be weakened by medicines such as steroids, which are taken for a number of different conditions like asthma, chronic lung disease (COPD), and lupus; anti-rejection medicines that are taken after organ transplants; or powerful chemotherapy used to fight cancer. If your immune system is down, the functions of your healing cells are compromised, thus preventing tissue repair. There are many other diseases that cause a weakened immune system like lupus, rheumatoid arthritis, and HIV.

Multiple Chronic Illnesses

Your body only has so much energy available and, if most of that energy is used constantly to fight chronic illness, less is available to repair skin damage. Furthermore, when there is limited energy available, your body slows down all of its processes in order to save energy. In other words, your metabolism slows down to make up for the constant losses. The stress that your body experiences from long-term illness also causes decreased production of proteins that are required to fight injury. You are using all of your protein, fat, and energy stores to fight the illness, and your body is unable to replace them. This can lead to a vicious cycle that is hard to stop without medical and nutritional intervention.

Dehydration and Excessively Dry Skin

The best environment for successful skin repair is slightly moist. Your body needs water to carry nutrients in and out of cells, as well as deliver oxygen to them. Skin cells cannot regenerate without the proper amount of moisture. Dry skin is more likely to be injured and heal poorly. Dry skin experiences more friction, which, in turn, leads to abrasions and ulcers. Dry skin also does not have the same elasticity as moisturized skin, so it can't stretch and adjust when it is pulled. Some people are born with a tendency to have dry skin, but often, dry skin is due to poor water intake, medications, extreme temperatures, bathing too frequently, products or chemicals applied to the skin, and poor diet.

▼ 4 ▼

Prevention of Pressure Ulcers

The simplest way to prevent bed sores is to not allow prolonged pressure on any particular area of the body, but every caregiver knows that is easier said than done. Most sources say that a bedbound person should be turned every two hours, and hospitals and long-term care facilities use a number of different turning protocols based on this time frame to ensure patient safety and to minimize the risk of a pressure injury.

However, there is little evidence to back up this custom. In reality, when your loved one is sitting upright or in a wheelchair, they should shift their weight every fifteen to thirty minutes. Standard wheelchairs are built so that both hips and knees rest at a 90-degree angle. But given that lots of health conditions like arthritis, scoliosis, muscle weakness, or partial paralysis limit your loved one's ability to safely achieve this position, pressure ends up on bony surfaces like the tailbone, ischia (the sit bones at the center of both sides of the buttocks), and hips.

If possible, buy a wheelchair with an adjustable back rest and place a pressure redistribution cushion (often called a Roho) in the wheelchair to help reduce the risk of injury. The cost of these cushions ranges from $350 to $400 but it may be covered by your insurer. Meanwhile, leg amputees may not have thigh bones that are long enough to support their body to sit upright in a wheelchair at 90 degrees, which places increased pressure and weight on the sit bones. So, they definitely need a pressure-distributing seat cushion.

To make a turning schedule tailored to your loved one's needs, test how long it takes for their skin to turn red when left

in the same position. Your turning schedule should be about thirty minutes less
than whatever that time is. For instance, if
it takes an hour and thirty minutes for the
skin to discolor, then you should turn your
loved every hour.

Many caregivers naturally think that it's
a good idea to use pillows under their loved
one's feet to keep their heels off the bed and
to prevent pressure ulcers. Unfortunately,
as we mentioned in the introduction, even
pillows can cause bed sores. In order to

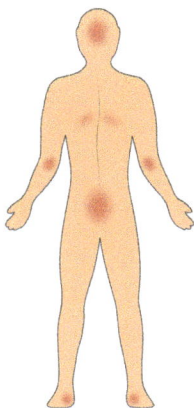

Pressure ulcer
dangerous body area

position the heels properly, nothing should be touching them except air. So, if pillows are going to be used, they must be placed underneath the knees and calves, which have more cushion from fat and muscle, compared to the heel. These areas can withstand more pressure.

Caregivers must also be careful not to damage fragile skin while moving their loved ones. When you change bed linen or move your loved one from one place to another (i.e., from a wheelchair to bed), you must actually lift them up off of the surface during the transfer. Do not slide or drag them from one surface to the next, which increases the risk of shearing their fragile skin and developing a chronic wound. Raising them up before you move them reduces the chances of such injuries.

Another important factor that requires focused attention is keeping the skin on the buttocks and genital region clean and free of urine and stool. This can be quite labor-intensive and is one of the most challenging aspects of caring for a loved one at home, especially if they don't move well. Prolonged exposure to excessive moisture from both stool and urine alters the pH of the skin, weakening it and making it swell. The skin then becomes more prone to injury from simple things like shearing when you slide your loved one from one surface to another, as well as to irritation (inflammation) and infection.

You might have heard of the term heat rash for patients with incontinence who develop rashes in the diaper area. The formal name of this rash is moisture-associated dermatitis, or MASD. MASD is not the same as a pressure ulcer, but when this inflammation of the skin is present, pressure ulcers are more likely to occur. It's important to know the difference between an early pressure ulcer and MASD, because they are treated differently. MASD causes itching and burning of the skin, which then looks red and inflamed and is warm to the touch. Unlike pressure wounds, which have sharp, distinct borders, the borders of MASD are hard to really define. However, you may notice little red dots along the borders of MASD; these are called satellite lesions and are signs of a fungal infection. That's why MASD responds to antifungal creams and powders, but pressure wounds do not.

Practically speaking, the best way to prevent MASD is to change diapers frequently, to cleanse the skin after each stool, and to apply barrier cream to the diaper region daily. When cleaning the affected area, do not rub the skin back and forth. Use a moist, unscented wipe and gently clean in one direction, front to back. Do not use regular washcloths because they are abrasive to the fragile skin in the diaper region. Instead, use disposable cloths that are made for incontinence care. Also, do *not* use scented baby wipes.

Traditional soaps are also not ideal for cleaning the skin of those who are incontinent. Most soaps are alkaline, meaning they raise the pH of the skin. Bacteria thrives on higher pH and makes the outer protective layer of the skin less effective. Once again, excess moisture from urine and stool penetrate the barrier and the skin gets swollen and more prone to injury. If possible, use a cleanser that can be sprayed on the skin and does not have to be rinsed/wiped off.

After bathing or cleaning, keep the skin properly moisturized. This will reduce itching and prevent incidental injury from scratching. Moisturized skin can also resist damage from trauma and repair itself more easily. As mentioned before, hydration is critical in the renewal process and to help the skin perform its number one duty: to act as a barrier to harmful bacteria and other germs. Gentle, emollient-based products give the best long-lasting moisture. Choose products without heavy perfumes to minimize the potential for irritation.

Chapter

5

Nutrition and Wound Care

Your loved one needs proper nutrition to heal their wounds. A malnourished person does not take in the protein, fat, carbohydrate, vitamins, and minerals needed to maintain healthy, robust skin or to repair skin injury. Though obese individuals eat more regularly, they often have protein calorie malnutrition because they are likely eating processed foods rather than healthy, nutrient-rich foods with vitamins and minerals. Regardless of the one's conditions, lack of vitamins can cause deep cracks in the skin, rashes, dryness, flakiness, and itching.

Proper protein intake is an absolute must in order to get wounds to heal. This is because just about every system in your body is made of protein. Hormones are made of protein. Our skin cells, muscles, and bones are made of protein. All of the cells in our immune system are made of protein, and it is our immune system that is most involved in protecting us from injury and then repairing any damage that might happen. Without the proper amount of nutrients in our diet, our skin cannot protect and defend itself from trauma, which makes it more prone to injury from everyday occurrences. Some great sources of protein include eggs, dairy, meat, beans, chicken, peanut butter, almond butter, and fish.

If you feel like your loved one is not eating and drinking enough (i.e., eating less than 50% of their meals), you must share this information with their health care team so they may refer you to a nutritionist. A nutritionist can look at your family member's typical diet and figure out their deficits, while factoring in health conditions such as kidney disease, diabetes, kidney stones, blood clots, high blood pressure, and heart failure that will affect their ideal diet. For instance, people who have chronic kidney disease must watch the amount of protein they eat. Diabetics must watch the type of sugar and starches they eat. People with heart disease or high cholesterol must watch their salt and fat intake. A nutritionist is trained to take all these special requirements into account. Together, you can craft a plan to increase your family member's nutrient and calorie intake based on foods that they like and will actually eat, all while being careful not to worsen any other health conditions.

One of the best things you can do to encourage better nutrition for your loved one is to simply feed them what they want while creatively sneaking in extra calories and nutrients. Don't force them to eat okra if you know they don't like it; instead, add nutrients to the foods they will actually eat. Sneak some extra vegetables into their spaghetti sauce. Put butter on their vegetables if they're underweight. Add tasteless, powdered fiber like Benefiber to any sauce, water, or juice. Add ground flax seeds to their cereal. Increase protein intake by adding powdered milk to soups, casseroles, mashed potatoes, and pudding. Chances are, they're not watching you prepare the food!

Also consider supplementing the diet with nutritional shakes such as Boost, Ensure, and Glucerna. These companies offer coupons on their respective websites and Boost (made by Nestle) has lots of recipes to help you mix these supplements into your loved one's regular food.

Chapter

▼ 6 ▼

Old School Remedies

Much of what most people know about treating rashes, sores, and skin injuries, we learned from our parents and grandparents. Some of these practices may be safe but are actually unhelpful. Other practices are straight up harmful. We'll discuss some of those popular home remedies.

Practice #1: Rubbing alcohol

Rubbing alcohol has no place on healthy skin! I know, I know, I know: your mother used it on your scrapes and bruises all the time when you were little to "clean it." You probably still remember how much it burned when she did. That is because rubbing alcohol kills everything in its path. You will not just kill any dirt and germs in the wound, but also healthy tissue. But doctors and nurses use alcohol pads all the time before you get a shot—how bad could it be? A simple wipe of alcohol is okay to reduce the activity of bacteria on your skin before you introduce a foreign object. But pouring alcohol into an open wound? Out of the question.

Practice #2: Hydrogen peroxide

See above. An excellent disinfectant that has no place in the care of damaged skin. It has actually been shown to *delay* healing time, likely because it kills fibroblasts that help repair injured skin. It has also been shown to disrupt capillaries, which are tiny blood vessels that supply blood to your skin. If you disrupt blood flow to the skin's cells, it cannot renew itself. Plus, those capillaries form granulation tissue, which is also critical in the process of wound healing.

Practice #3: Duct tape or household tape

Never use these to cover wounds! You can literally rip your loved one's healthy skin right off. Even if somehow you managed to remove these products without tearing the skin, the adhesive used on these types of tape is very likely to irritate the skin, causing itching, burning, and rashes,

Practice #4: Vinegar

Overall, the use of vinegar for wound healing is frowned upon in the medical community. Vinegar slows down the growth of new skin cells in the wound, a process called epithelialization. Once again, this popular antiseptic not only kills bacteria, but also kills fibroblasts, even when it is diluted down to ¼ of its original strength. It also kills another important type of cells in the healing process: neutrophils, or white blood cells that kill bacteria and other germs. When these guys don't work, harmful bacteria grow and infect wounds.

There's one exception in which case vinegar may be beneficial on a wound: when it is infected by bacteria called Pseudomonas aeruginosa. However, you cannot know that a wound is infected with Pseudomonas without having a proper wound culture performed by a doctor or nurse; so even though there is an exception to the rule, vinegar should still not be used without the supervision of a wound care professional. In other words, don't try this at home!

Practice #5: Betadine and mercurochrome

Like peroxide, betadine has been found to actually impair the healing process because—you guessed it—in addition to killing bacteria, it kills fibroblasts. Betadine is great for keeping bacteria away from dead tissue like eschar that is frequently seen on the heels, but it should not be applied to open wounds.

Mercurochrome is another "old school" remedy that used to be applied on minor scrapes and bruises. It fell out of favor in many countries because of its mercury content and has not been distributed in the U.S. with mercury as one of its ingredients since 1998 due to concerns of potential poisoning. In case you need more reasons not to use it, here are a couple more: it stings when applied, sometimes causes a rash, and also interferes with wound healing.

Practice #6: Vicks

There is no shortage of articles that encourage the use of Vicks to heal wounds. But even the product manufacturer's instructions discourage this use. The active ingredients in Vicks are camphor, eucalyptus oil, and menthol, while the inactive ingredients include petrolatum and turpentine oil. Petrolatum itself is actually a key treatment in wound care that is safe and effective when used in the right setting and perhaps that's the reason why it has been recommended in non-medical settings. However, petrolatum is only one of many ingredients listed in Vicks, and the others can have potential side effects such as a burning sensation, skin irritation, redness, and rash.

Chapter

7

Does the Wound Need Air?

One of the most common mistakes that I see caregivers and patients make is removing dressings from a wound because they think it "needs air." Once again, wounds heal the fastest when they are given a slightly moist environment. Each step of the wound-healing process requires water. When a wound is too dry, a scab forms, which can block new skin cells from growing. Scabs are not a sign of healing. They are the remnants of dead skin cells and debris.

The second most common mistake is changing dressings too often. Best practices in wound care include changing dressings as little as is necessary. This is because, every time you remove a dressing, you traumatize the would and also risk damaging the surrounding, healthy skin. Most wounds do not need to be changed multiple times a day, given that most wound care products require a certain amount of time to work properly: some only need to be changed every two to three days, while others have active ingredients that only last for twenty-four hours. If you change the dressing more frequently than recommended, you stop the healing actions of the dressings before they have fully had a chance to work.

Lastly, but just as importantly, dressing changes are uncomfortable for the patient. You can reduce your loved one's discomfort by not changing dressings multiple times daily. This is an area that's important to discuss with your wound care team. Make sure you tell the doctors and nurses if a certain type of dressing or regimen they prescribe doesn't actually work for you and be sure to state the reasons why. There are literally hundreds of wound-care dressing and products to choose from. Regardless of fancy advertising, the best product is the one you will use properly. Share your concerns so that you reach a plan of care *together* and troubleshoot issues before they become a huge problem. The key to effective wound care is finding the right plan for the caregiver and his or her loved one.

8

How to Choose the Best Dressing

If there are thousands of wound care products available, how are you supposed to choose the right one? It really boils down to the level of moisture in the wound. Wounds that produce a lot of drainage (called exudate) need dressings that can absorb that moisture and wick it away from the skin's surface. Wounds that are dry need products that will add just the right amount of moisture. It is critical to keep the wound slightly moist in order to promote the growth of new skin cells. If the dressing creates too much moisture in the wound bed, the skin and tissue become way too wet and macerated. Macerated tissue is weak, fragile, and prone to injury; you can hurt it just by touching it. Like the Goldilocks fairytale, you must get the moisture level *just right.*

The second characteristic that dictates what type of dressing is best for a wound is the type of tissue is in the wound bed. Is there new skin growing? Is it bright pink and grainy/bumpy? Is it black and smelly? Is it tan/yellow? Can you see muscle, bone, or tendons inside the wound? Remember epithelial and bright pink granulation tissue are good. Black, yellow, or tan colored tissue (eschar and slough) is not.

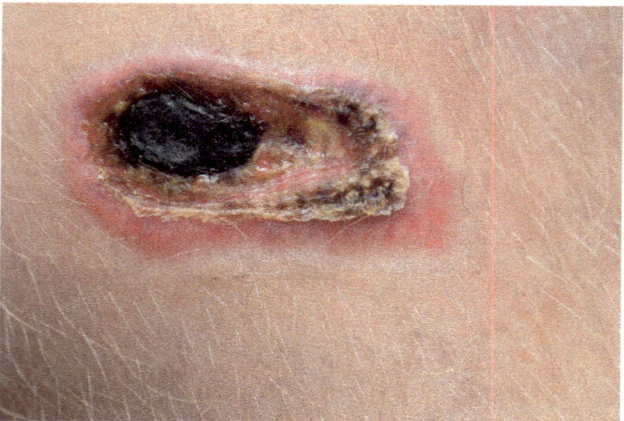

Epithelial tissue is new skin cells that grow in the wound. These cells are what we work so hard to get. They grow over the layer of granulation tissue, usually from the outside or perimeter of the wound toward the inside. Occasionally, they show up randomly dispersed in the center of a wound for no apparent reason. New epithelial tissue is fragile and must not be disturbed by things like friction, exposure to bandage tape/adhesives, and frequent or unnecessary dressing changes.

Granulation tissue is formed by connective tissue and new capillaries growing in a wound. The capillaries form a lattice-like structure, which looks like fine bumps to the naked eye and also looks thicker than normal skin. Healthy granulation tissue is bright pink/slightly red and bleeds easily. Pale granulation tissue that does not bleed when irritated may be a sign that the wound bed is not healthy.

Slough is dead or dying tissue (necrotic) in a wound bed. It comes from debris that

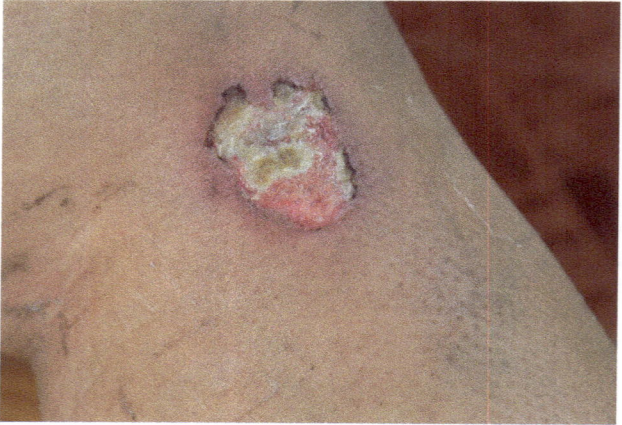

is left from dead skin cells, pus, white blood cells, bacteria, and other proteins. It usually looks moist, sometimes stringy, and is pale yellow or tan in color. Sometimes, it is hard to tell the difference between slough and fat because of their similar color and because slough is usually stuck to the tissue underneath it.

Eschar is black or dark brown in color and often very thick, almost like leather. Eschar is made of dead or dying tissue and sometimes has an odor. Eschar is often found on the heels that develop pressure ulcers. It may be tempting to pick at the eschar on a loved one's wound, much like you might pick an ordinary scab. However, this is dangerous idea because you have no idea how deep the dead tissue goes and no idea what's underneath it. The tissue underneath the eschar may bleed, and you may not be able to stop the bleeding. Sometimes, there is also a collection of pus underneath, which you may not be prepared to handle.

Slough and eschar in a wound are a problem. Both attract bacteria to the wound and can lead to heavy colonization or frank infection. Most often, slough impedes wound healing, and it must be removed. Eschar, in particular, is a sign of tissue death. Healthy, new tissue cannot grow until the dead tissue is removed, a process called debridement. Wound debridement can be accomplished with a topical medication and/or manually with gauze or sharp instruments. Wound debridement definitely requires the training and expertise of a wound care professional.

A Brief Summary of Wound Dressings and Therapies

There are a variety of wound care products and dressings available on the market. They range from simple, dry dressings like gauze or ABD pads (thick, cushioned, rectangular shaped bandages) all the way to highly specialized skin substitutes that cost hundreds to thousands of dollars. Most wounds will require more than just a dry dressing like gauze, an absorptive pad, and tape, since these products pull moisture from the wound. The fluid in the wound travels from the skin onto to the dry dressing and stays there unless you put some type of topical ointment on the skin to keep this from happening. Always remember: the best environment for a wound is a slightly moist one.

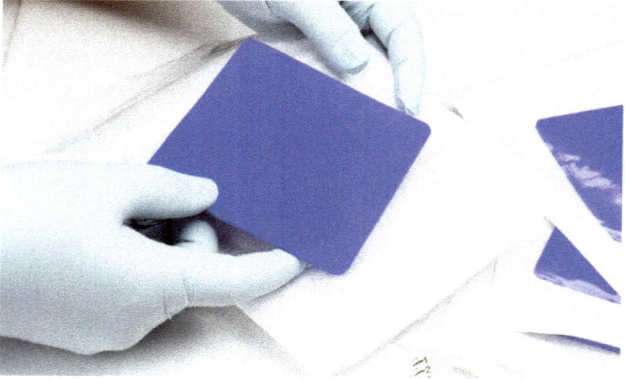

The following are the most common types of wound dressings, ointments, and treatments available for wound healing:

- *Hydrogel:* this is a water-based gel that adds moisture to a wound. It is best used on wounds that produce very little fluid. It is one of the least expensive treatments available and is very easy to use. You can apply the gel directly to the wound using a cotton tip applicator (commonly known as a Q-tip) or you can apply the gel to gauze and secure with tape or use bordered gauze. Wounds treated with hydrogel are typically changed daily.

- *Collagen:* this protein is responsible for your skin being plump and strong, and is used as a wound dressing when we try to get granulation tissue to form. It helps bring in all of the proteins that are needed to help new skin grow and supports the body as it gets rid of the proteins that prolong inflammation.

  Collagen comes in many different forms like paste, powder, gels, and even embedded in alginate. Regardless of which form you choose, you will have to cover the collagen with another dry dressing like gauze or a bordered foam. Wounds dressed with collagen are often changed every two to three days ideally, but some collagen dressings can be left in place up to an entire week.

- *Alginates:* this thick, felt-like dressing is made partly from seaweed, and is best used in wounds that produce a lot of fluid and are too wet. The seaweed is very absorptive, holding a great deal of extra fluid away from the skin.

  Alginate must be changed depending on how much fluid the wound makes. Very wet wounds must be changed once or twice daily, while others may only need changes every other day. Ask your wound care team for advice if you are unsure. Occasionally, alginates can get stuck to the wound bed as the wound dries. This can cause pain when it is removed, so add some saline or water to the dressing before you try to remove it to prevent discomfort.

- *Silver:* known for its anti-microbial properties, silver is used a lot in wound care. It is available as a gel or foam and is also embedded in alginate. Silver is particularly helpful in wounds that are very wet, highly infected, or are heavily colonized with bacteria. If the wound is dry, silver gel is useful in adding moisture and fighting bacterial overgrowth.

- *Honey:* medical-grade honey is popular in wound care because of its ability to fight bacteria, remove dead tissue, and add a bit of moisture to the wound. Wounds treated with medical-grade honey only need to be changed every three days because it takes time for the honey to work. If you change the wound too often, you will not reap the benefits.

- *Iodosorb:* this iodine-based product helps reduce the presence of bacteria in a wound and reduces inflammation. Iodosorb comes in a gel form and needs to be applied directly to a dry dressing and then onto the wound. This dressing needs to be changed depending on what's going on inside the wound, but is usually changed anywhere between one and three days. This dressing does not require a doctor's prescription and can be purchased online through sites like Amazon, often at a cheaper price than what you will find in a brick and mortar pharmacy. *Do not use Iodosorb if your loved one has an iodine allergy!*

- *Santyl:* This ointment is made of the enzyme collagenase, which breaks down slough and eschar. It is the only medication of its kind on the marketplace. Other wound care products can reduce slough, but they do so using a different method that takes longer.

  It should be applied directly on the wound in a layer that is nickel thick and covered with a moistened gauze to activate its slough-fighting power. If the wound already makes a lot of fluid on its own, then a dry dressing can be used because the wound's fluid will be enough to activate the enzyme. Wounds that are treated with Santyl must be changed daily since the active ingredients work best within twenty-four hours.

- *Foam:* this is good for absorbing excess fluid and keeping the wound slightly moist. It also protects the injured skin from the trauma of dressing changes. From my experience, foam is favored by many wound care providers when there is hypergranulation tissue in a wound, which won't close as fast or may not close at all until the extra tissue is removed.

- *Hydrofera Blue:* this foam-based dressing is ideal for wounds that produce mild to moderate drainage. It also has anti-inflammatory and anti-bacterial properties that make it a great weapon in a variety of wound healing. It comes in squared pieces of foam that have a bright bluish-purple color.

- *Skin substitutes:* these are incredibly expensive, highly specialized dressings that are full of cells harvested from the placenta at childbirth and/or the foreskin of the penis after circumcision. These cells are full of high growth potential, more than any functioning adult cells. The tissue is cleansed, and the growth factors are separated out and formulated into a dressing. This dressing can only be used in a wound care center or hospital setting. I've seen them work wonders when multiple other products have failed, but they are only used on patients that meet certain criteria, and they require very specific care in order to work.

- *Negative Pressure Wound Therapy (NPWT) aka "Wound Vacs:"* This therapy is effective in treating large wounds, deep wounds, and wounds that produce a lot of drainage. The negative pressure sucks drainage out of the wound, away from the skin, and into a canister. NPWT also stimulates the growth of granulation tissue and pulls wound edges together, which closes it and fills dead space caused by under-mining.

A big challenge when using NPWT is keeping a good seal. If the vac is not properly sealed onto the skin, the device shuts off. This can happen if the skin around the wound is wet or oily from lotion, cleansing agents, etc. when the device is applied. Also, too often people just leave the vac covering in place even when the device is not working properly, and they also don't change the dressing; this causes the wound to get too wet, smelly, and usually larger in size.

If, for some reason, the machine is not working, remove it from the wound and cover it with a dry dressing like foam or alginate. Then, call your wound care professional to let them know that the vac is not working and to make a plan for what dressing you should use in place of the vac. The wound must be looked at by someone on the team at the earliest available appointment to prevent a setback in healing.

Chapter

▼ 10

Hyperbaric Oxygen Therapy: It's Not Just for Divers

Hyperbaric oxygen therapy (HBO) is the practice of breathing air that has a higher concentration of oxygen than the normal air that we breathe. The air is pressurized to achieve this state, and that is why you have to sit or lie in a special chamber while that pressure is safely increased for treatment. When we breathe in this air, that higher concentration of oxygen gets carried in our blood and delivered to all of our organs and tissues, thus improving healing.

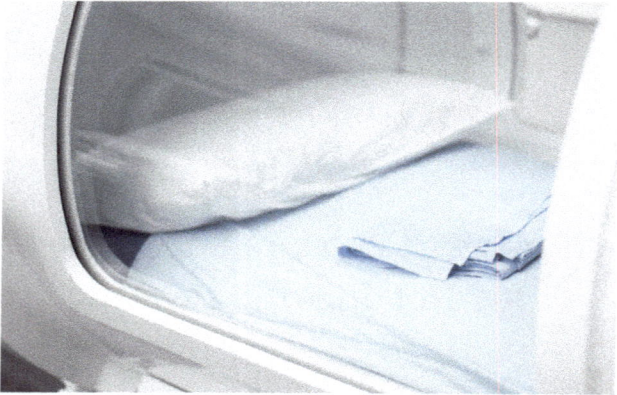

Most people and even physicians have never heard of HBO, outside of possibly knowing that it helps deep-sea divers from getting "the bends." However, it has multiple uses in medicine, such as preventing damage from radiation in patients with cancer of the mouth or throat who undergo therapy. For patients being treated with radiation for cancer in the prostate or cervix, HBO repairs damage that sometimes occurs to the surrounding organs in the pelvis, such as the bladder. It has also been proven to improve outcomes for diabetic ulcers, arterial ulcers, and chronic bone infections called osteomyelitis, as well as for failing skin grafts and flaps, and carbon monoxide poisoning. HBO can mean the difference between amputation and restoration; I have seen it literally save lives and limbs.

To receive the therapy, you lie in a special chamber shaped like a cylinder for about an hour every day, five times per week usually for four weeks at a minimum. There is no pain. Your ears may pop at the beginning and end of treatment like when you're on an airplane taking off or landing. In the chamber, you can take a nap, listen to music, or watch TV while the concentrated air heals your body.

In many ways, HBO really is like magic, but it doesn't work for everything, and there are some people who should not receive it, such as those who have untreated cataracts and certain lung diseases. Unfortunately, there is not enough evidence yet that HBO will improve pressure ulcers. But if your loved one has a pressure ulcer on the legs, ankle, or foot, as well as diabetes, they may still qualify for the therapy. If you don't ask, you will never know. As I mentioned at the beginning of the book, I have seen countless patients undergo amputations that might have been able to be prevented if they had been offered alternatives like this.

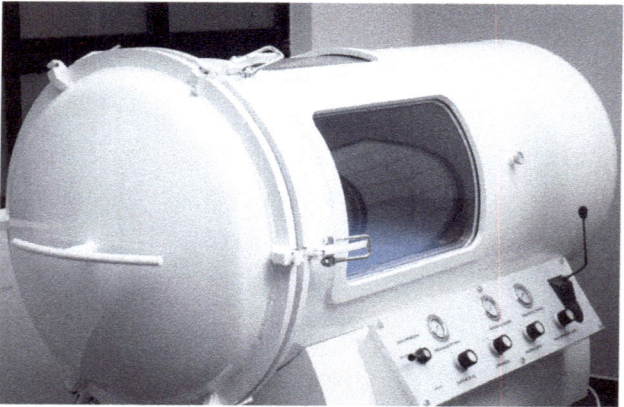

Please ask your doctor about this therapy if your loved one has an unhealed wound and/or bone infection and the medical team has mentioned the possible need for amputation. Remember that most physicians and nurses are not trained in wound care and definitely not hyperbaric medicine. Not all wound care centers offer it. If time allows, push for this option and get a second opinion from a wound care center that offers HBO before you allow your loved one to undergo an amputation. HBO is covered on most insurance plans including Medicare and Medicaid.

Chapter 11

When to Ask for Help

Even if you don't know all the correct terminology or don't remember any of the technical aspects that have been covered in this book, you still have your gut instincts. Trust them. You know if your loved one is experiencing more pain than usual and if dressing changes are becoming more uncomfortable. You know when something doesn't look, feel, or smell right. You change the dressings day in and day out. You know what is and isn't working for you and your family.

Describe what you see as best you can and tell your wound care team what you are worried about. If you've been using the same type of dressing for several weeks and the wound is not getting better, speak up to your health care team. If your loved one has repeatedly been placed on antibiotics for a skin infection by their primary physician or nurse and the wound is not getting better, seek another opinion. Don't be afraid to ask for a referral to a wound care clinic.

At a dedicated wound care center, they have a war chest of options to treat wounds that most primary care physician or other health care provider won't have. If a wound needs to be cleaned up (debrided) at a wound care center, that procedure happens right at the bedside, whenever necessary. Oftentimes, no referral is needed to make an appointment at such a center. You can call the clinic and schedule an appointment yourself. Look for large, academic hospitals because they are most likely to have dedicated wound care centers.

Glossary of Terms

Acute: new or fresh; present less than 8 weeks

Artery: a vessel that carries oxygen-rich blood to all of our internal organs, skin, muscles, and bones in order to keep them alive.

Capillaries: tiny blood vessels that connect arteries and veins.

Cellulitis: bacterial infection of the skin and tissues beneath it.

Chronic: something that continues over time or a condition that keeps reoccurring. Wounds are considered to be chronic when they have not healed in four to eight weeks.

Collagen: a type of protein in the body that helps give our tissues like skin, bone, and cartilage their structure.

Colonized: refers to an increased number of bacteria living in a wound without the body mounting a response to fight them. More bacteria are present than normal, but not so many that the wound is infected. Colonization of a wound with bacteria can prevent it from healing.

Debridement: removing dead or otherwise unhealthy tissue from a wound. It can be accomplished with gauze, medicine, or a sharp instrument like a scalpel or specialized sharp instrument called a curette

Epithelium: another word for skin.

Epithelialization: the process in which new skin fills an area that used to be injured.

Eschar: thick, leathery, dead tissue, usually very dark brown or black in color.

Fibroblasts: proteins that are released during wound healing that create new collagen and other types of structural tissue like skin, cartilage, and bone.

Folliculitis: inflammation of the hair follicles that occurs due to trauma, infection, or exposure to a variety of substances.

Granulation tissue: new connective tissue that grows into a wound after the skin has been injured. It is made of collagen and tiny blood vessels and usually has a bright pink, lumpy-bumpy appearance.

Hemostasis: the process of getting bleeding to stop.

Hypergranulation tissue: new connective tissue that over-grows in a wound. It is thick, granular, and bleeds very easily. New skin cannot grow into a wound if it is blocked by this type of tissue.

Inflammation: the body's healing response to any kind of injury.

Macerated: describes skin that is too wet. It looks pale pink, grey, or white and is very fragile and easily injured.

Moisture-associated dermatitis: inflammation of the skin that is caused by too much moisture.

Negative Pressure Wound Therapy (NPWT): therapy that uses negative pressure to remove fluid and help close large or deep wounds.

Off-loading: the process of positioning the body to reduce pressure on a particular area.

Periwound: the area of healthy skin that surrounds a sore or ulcer.

Purulent: drainage or fluid that is filled with pus, thick yellow or green in color.

Regenerate: renew or re-grow.

Serous: drainage or fluid that is clear yellow.

Scar: fibrous tissue that replaces healthy skin after injury. It is not as healthy as intact skin and can cause pain.

Slough: a tan/yellow/ greyish-white colored collection of dead tissue cells and debris that collects in a wound. Sometimes, it prevents a wound from being able to heal.

Trauma: any type of injury like surgery, frostbite, burns, or punctures.

Ulcer: an area of skin that has layers missing due to injury; also known as a sore.

Vein: a vessel that carries blood away from our skin, muscles, bones, and internal organs and back toward the heart.

Venous insufficiency: a condition of the body in which the veins do not drain blood and send it back toward the heart as they are supposed to. This happens when the valves inside the veins stop working.

Wet to dry dressing: applying a bandage to a wet wound and then removing the dressing when the wound is dry. This is one of the oldest treatments in wound care, and it removes skin and causes pain as the dressing is removed.

Bibliography

Bigliardi, Paul Lorenz, et al. "Povidone Iodine in Wound Healing: A Review of Current Concepts and Practices." *International Journal of Surgery*, vol. 44, Aug. 2017, pp. 260–268., doi:10.1016/j.ijsu.2017.06.073.

Habif, Thomas P. *Skin Disease Diagnosis and Treatment*. Philadelphia: Elsevier Mosby, 2001.

Hess, Cathy Thomas. *Clinical Guide to Skin & Wound Care*. Philadelphia: Wolters Kluwer Health, 2008.

Morgan, Nancy. "What You Need to Know about Collagen Wound Dressings." *Wound Care Advisor*, 7 Apr. 2017, woundcareadvisor.com/what-you-need-to-know-about-collagen-wound-dressings/.

Nagoba, B.S., et al. "Acetic Acid Treatment of Pseudomonal Wound Infections: A

Review." *Journal of Infection and Public Health*, vol. 6, no. 6, 2013, pp. 410–415. doi:10.1016/j.jiph.2013.05.005.

Simon, Patrick. "Skin Wound Healing." *Medscape*, 20 Jan. 2016.

Sussman, Carrie. *Wound Care: A Collaborative Practice Manual for Health Professionals.* Philadelphia: Lippincott Williams & Wilkins, 2012.

"The Four Stages of Wound Healing." *WoundSource | Wound Care Products, Supplies, Dressings, Pressure Ulcers*, 28 Apr. 2016, www.woundsource.com/.

Wilson, and Clark. "'The Relationship Between Obesity and Wound Care' ." *Advanced Tissue*, 13 Aug. 2014.

Wilson, Joyce A., and Jan J. Clark. "Obesity: Impediment to Postsurgical Wound Healing."*Advances in Skin & Wound Care*, vol. 17, no. 8, Oct. 2004, pp. 426–432., doi:10.1097/00129334-200410000-00013.

Thank You!

I hope that this book has taught you some wound care basics that make you feel more comfortable and confident about the care you give. Refer back to it as often as necessary and use it as a reference to speak effectively with your wound care team.

If you have additional questions and would like additional coaching on caring for your loved one's wounds, please feel free to reach out to me via email at jjtaylor3md@gmail.com, via my website at Drjennifertaylor.com, or post your question to my Facebook page, @Drjennifertaylor.

About the Author

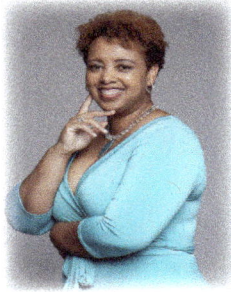

Dr. Jennifer Taylor is a board-certified family medicine physician, wound care specialist, entrepreneur, educator, author, and public speaker. She is also the owner and creator of Like Butter Baby, a line of natural body products designed to moisturize and heal damaged skin. She serves as a medical director for a major insurance company. Prior to this, she served as medical director of wound care and hyperbaric oxygen therapy for a nationally known wound care company, a team physician for a nationwide hospice care organization, and a physician advisor for a medical necessity compliance corporation.

Dr. Taylor completed her undergraduate degree at Northwestern University, and serves as an extended board member and as the chair of Pre-Health Student Based Initiatives for the Black Alumni Association at her alma mater. She is also a board member of a Cleveland, Ohio–based nonprofit foundation that is dedicated to providing educational, financial, and emotional support to at-risk adolescent men in urban communities.

Dr. Taylor earned her medical degree at University of Illinois College of Medicine and completed her residency at University Hospitals of Cleveland Case Medical Center. She resides in Chicago.

To connect, visit her website at
drjennifertaylor.com

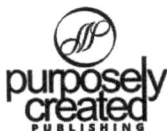

CREATING DISTINCTIVE BOOKS
WITH INTENTIONAL RESULTS

We're a collaborative group of creative masterminds
with a mission to produce high-quality books to position
you for monumental success in the marketplace.

Our professional team of writers, editors, designers,
and marketing strategists work closely together to ensure
that every detail of your book is a clear representation
of the message in your writing.

Want to know more?
Write to us at info@publishyourgift.com
or call (888) 949-6228

Discover great books, exclusive offers, and more at
www.PublishYourGift.com

Connect with us on social media

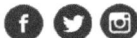

@publishyourgift